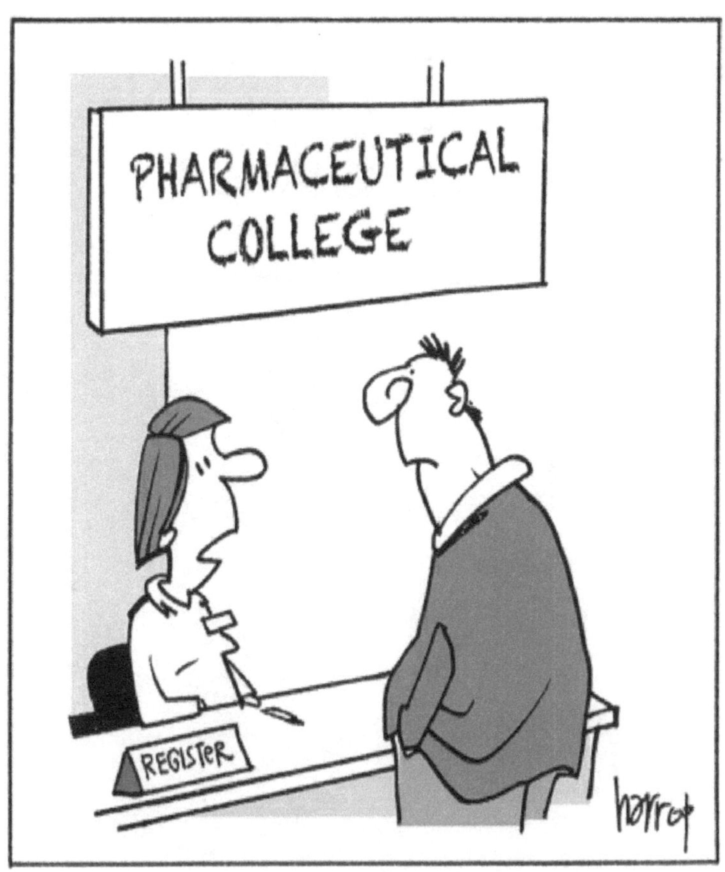

That's right - even if you already own a
white coat, we still expect you to take the course!

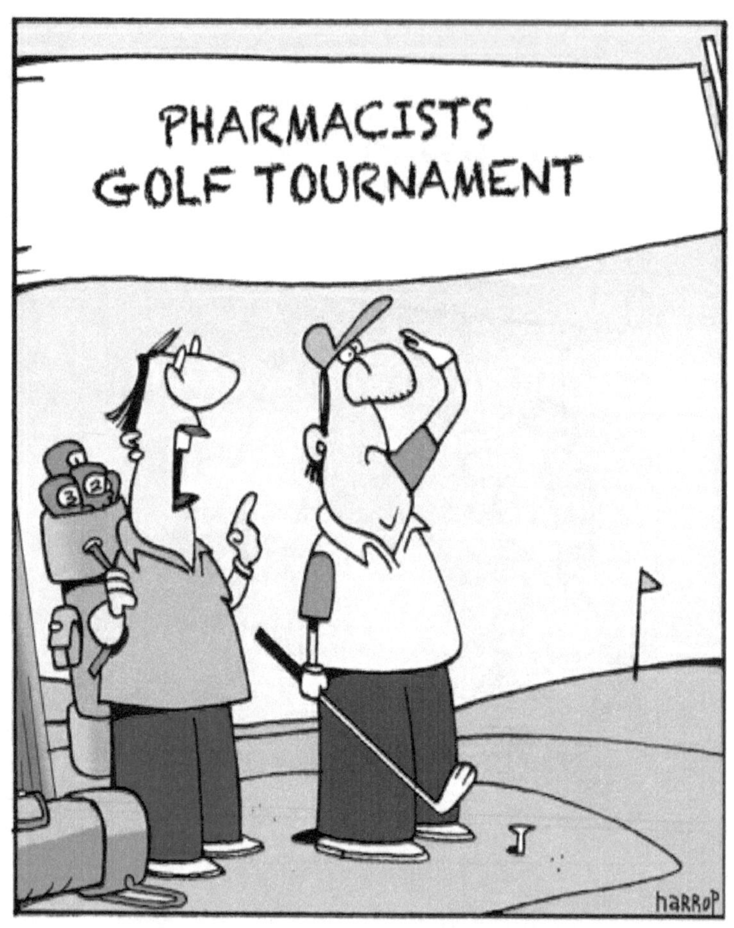

You've hit another pharmacist...
the good news is that he's wearing
a safety cap.

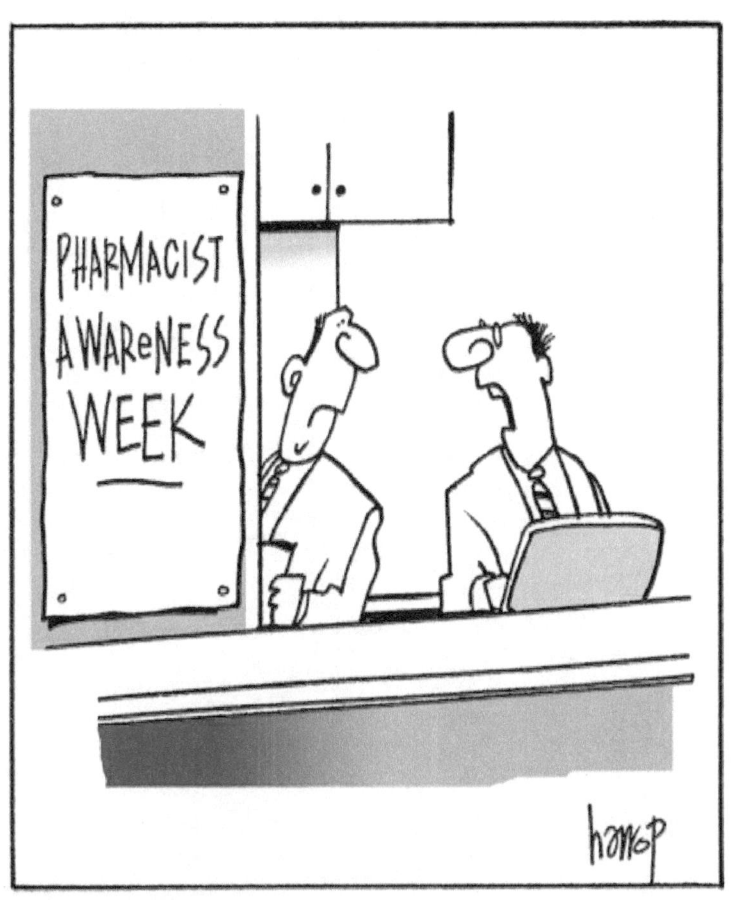

Of *COURSE* I'm aware of you, Waldren!
Now go back to work!

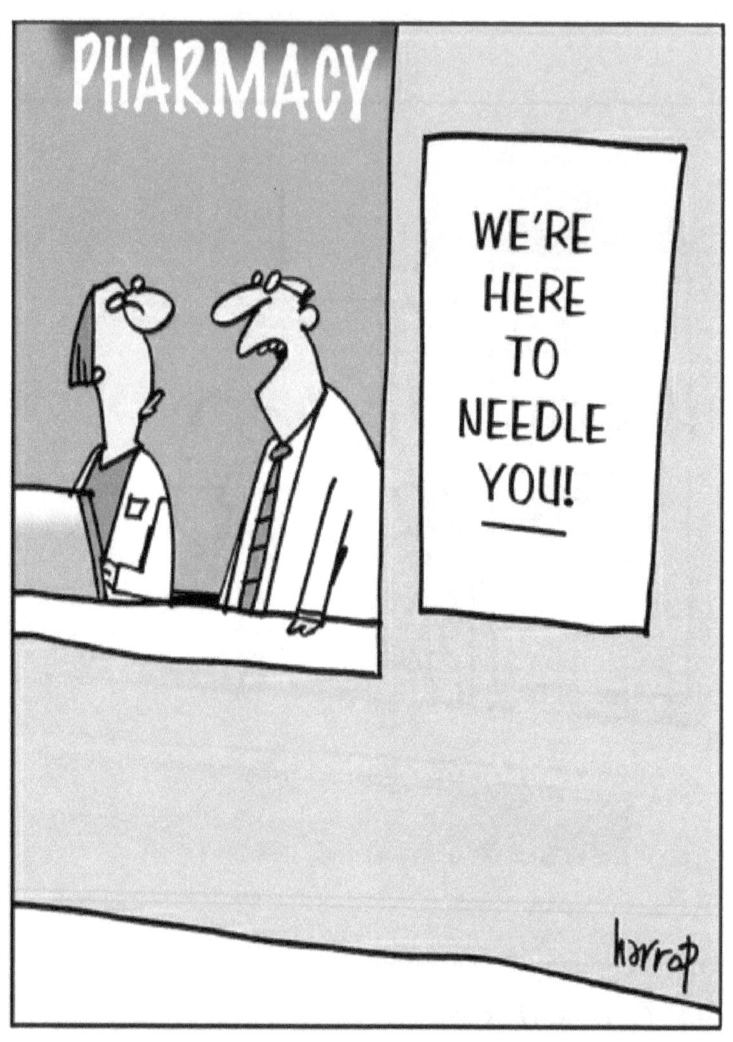

There's got to be a better way to say that
we give injections!

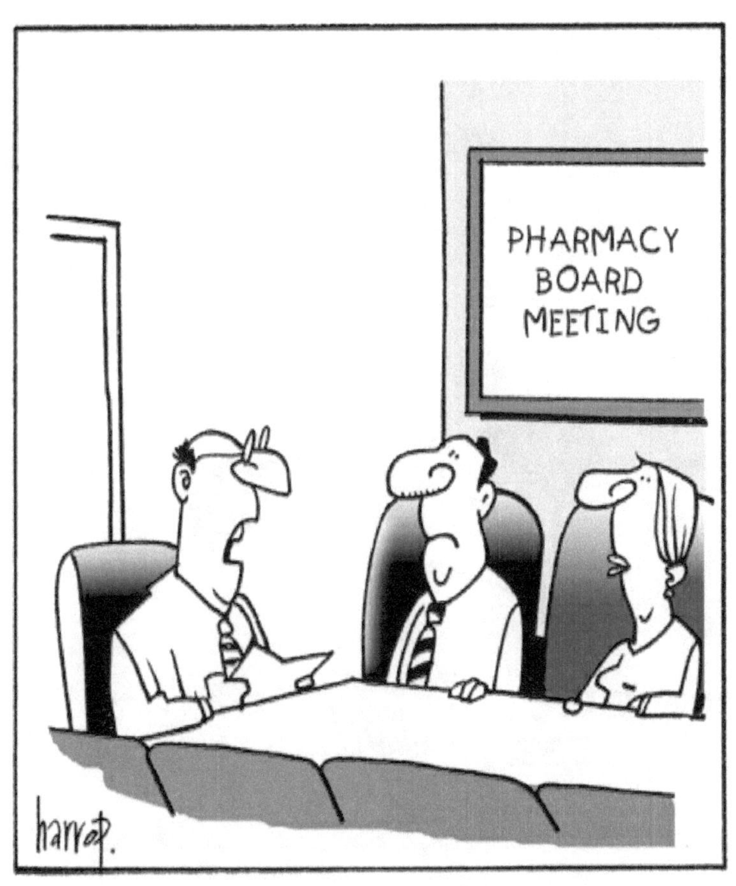

I don't care if we *ARE* on Twitter ...
stop calling me 'dude' ... !

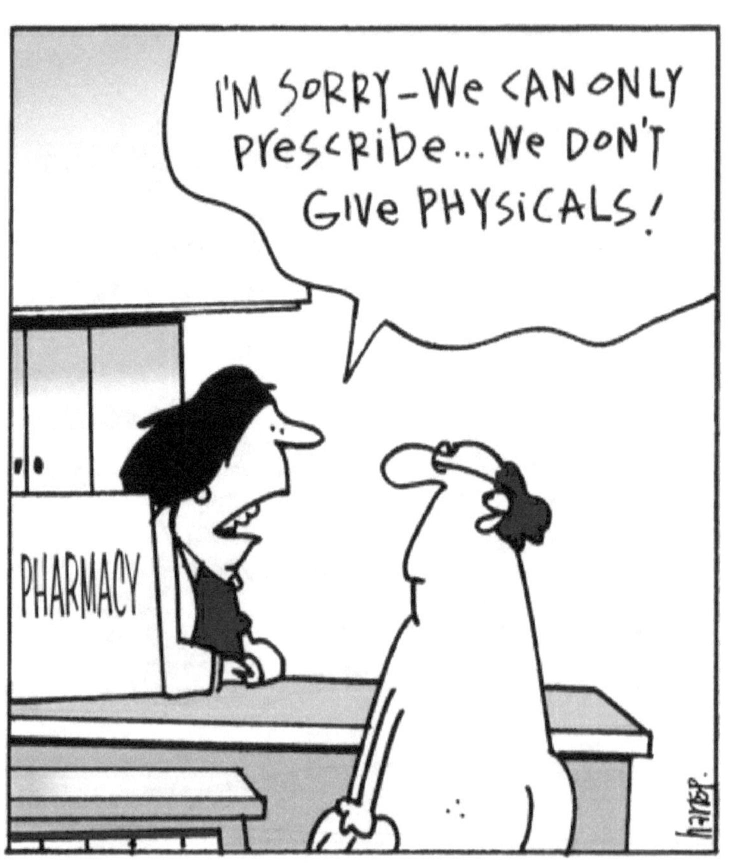

I'M SORRY—WE CAN ONLY PRESCRIBE...WE DON'T GIVE PHYSICALS!
PHARMACY

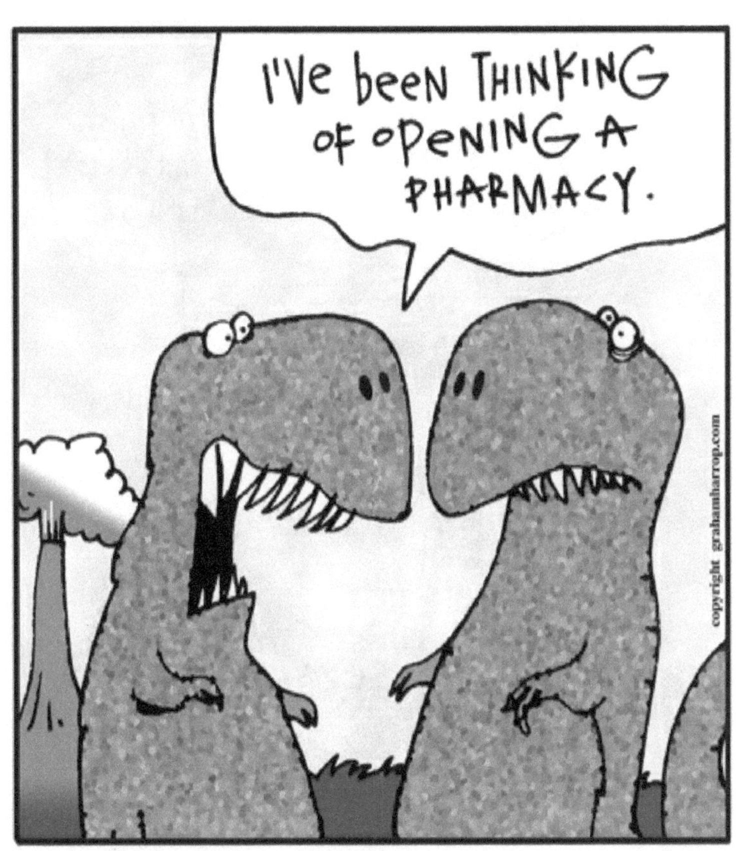

tyrannosaurus R$_x$

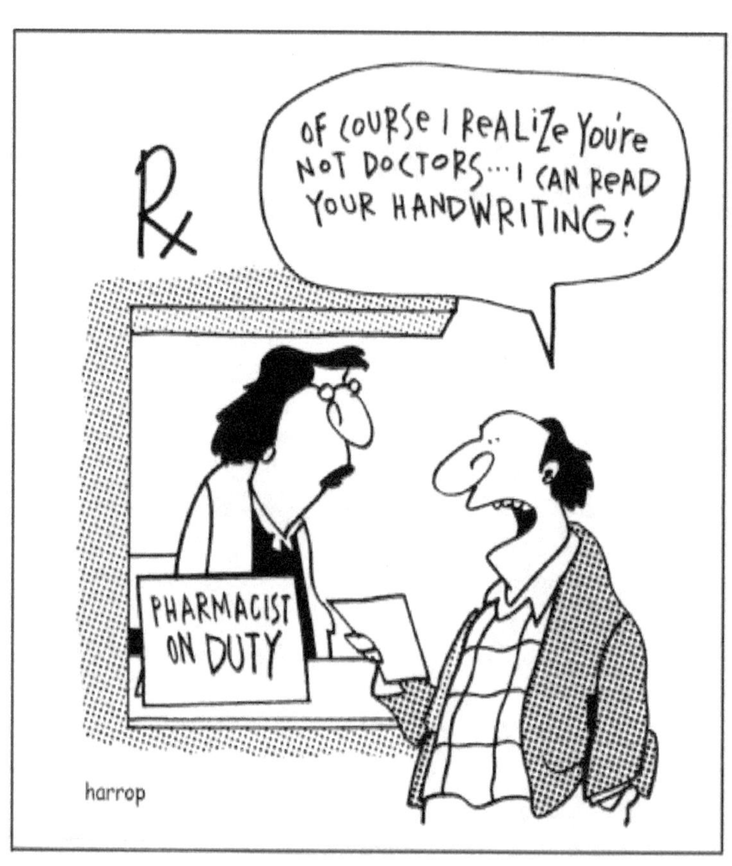

Rx
OF COURSE I REALIZE YOU'RE NOT DOCTORS... I CAN READ YOUR HANDWRITING!
PHARMACIST ON DUTY
harrop

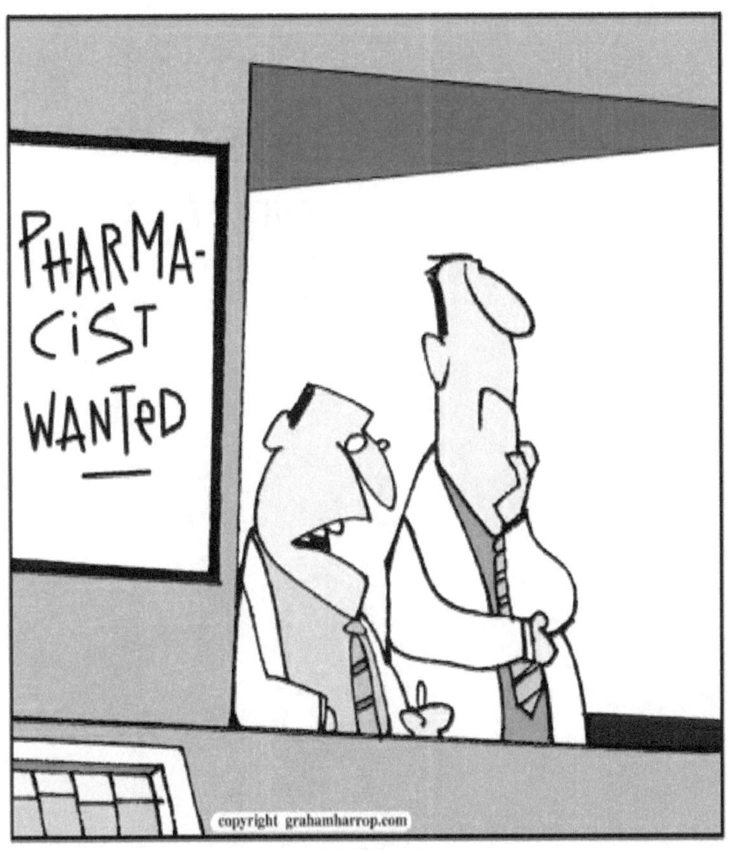

Maybe we should drop the: 'Leaps tall buildings in a single bound' requirement'.

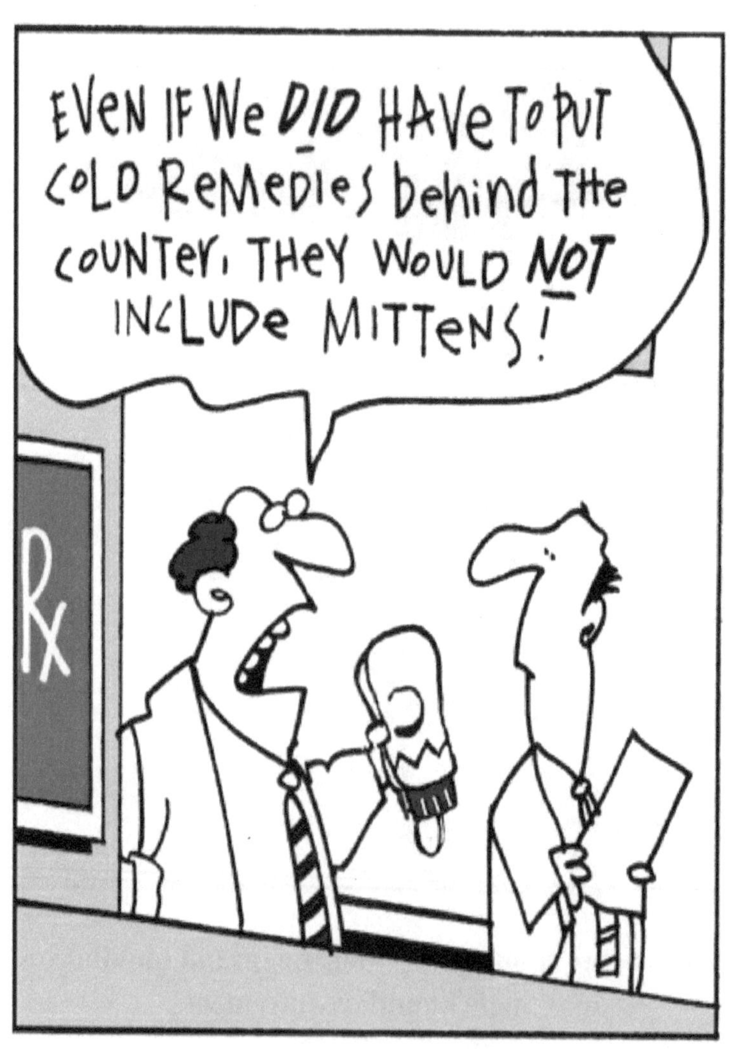
EVEN IF WE DID HAVE TO PUT COLD REMEDIES behind THE counter, THEY WOULD NOT INCLUDE MITTENS!
RX

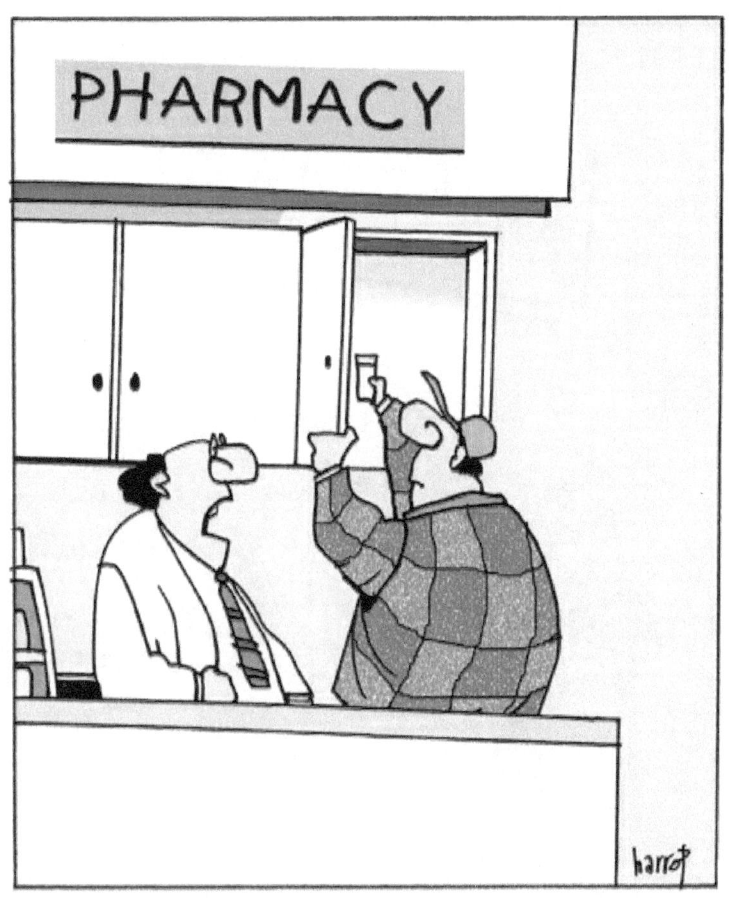

We're ALL in a hurry these days, Mr. Fossy,
but if you don't mind - I'll dispense
the medication!

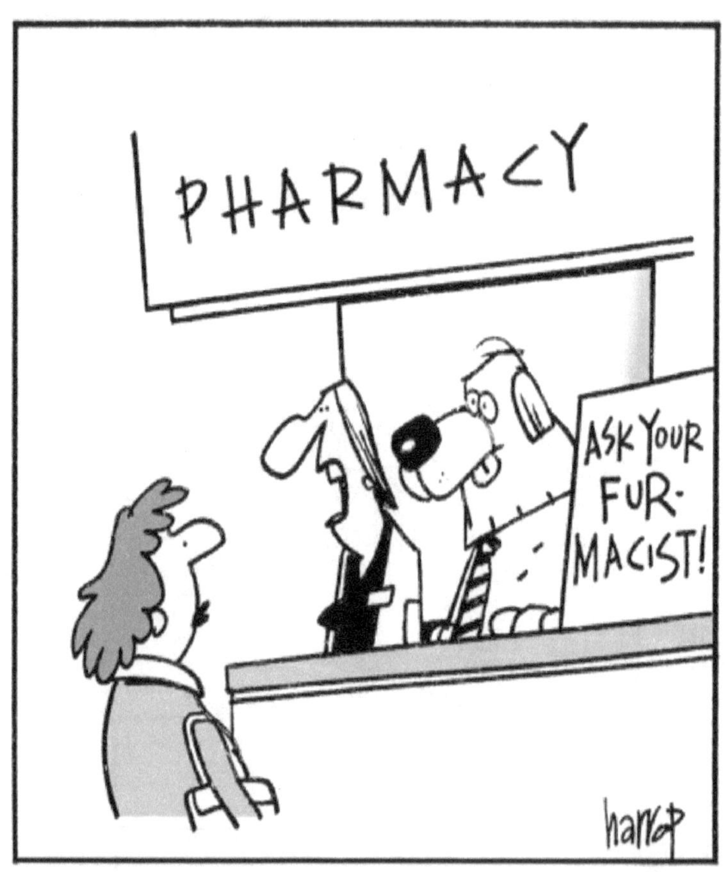

Ed's been wearing it ever since we started to dispense pet medication...!

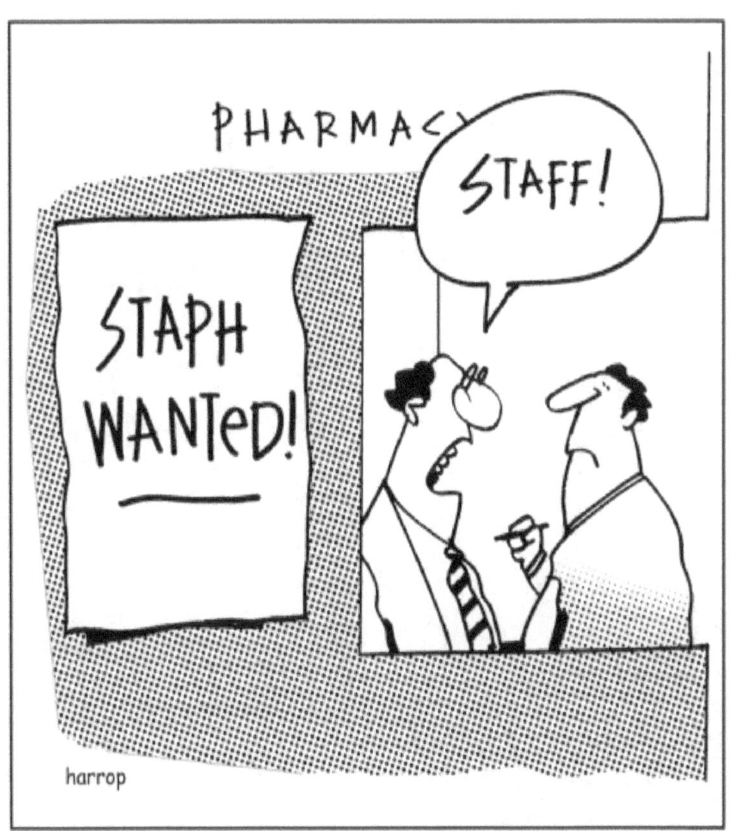

PHARMACY
STAFF!
STAPH
WANTED!
harrop

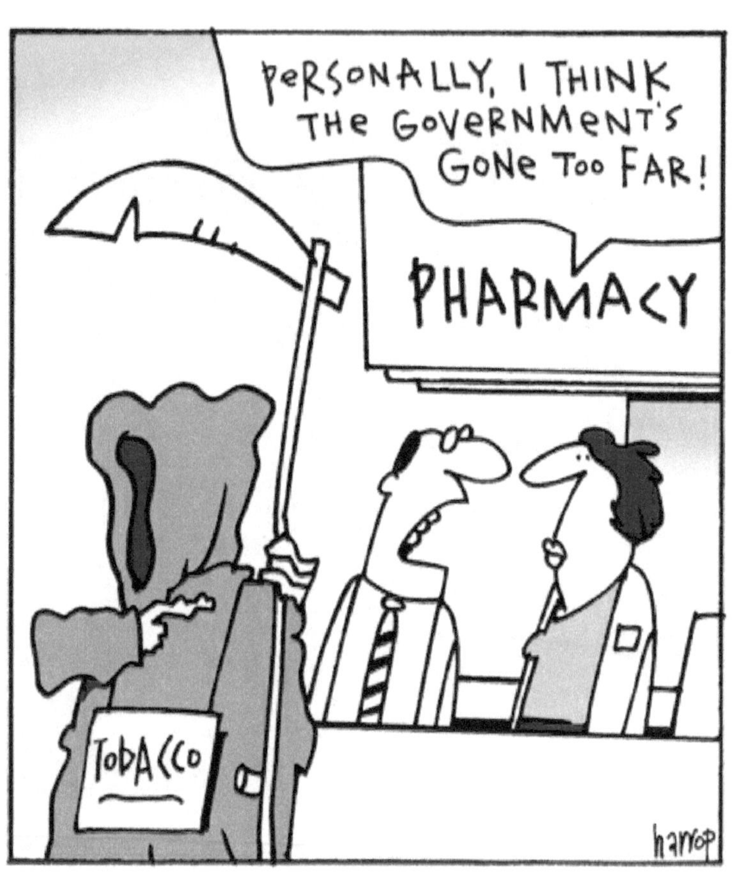

PERSONALLY, I THINK THE GOVERNMENT'S GONE TOO FAR!
PHARMACY
TOBACCO
harrop

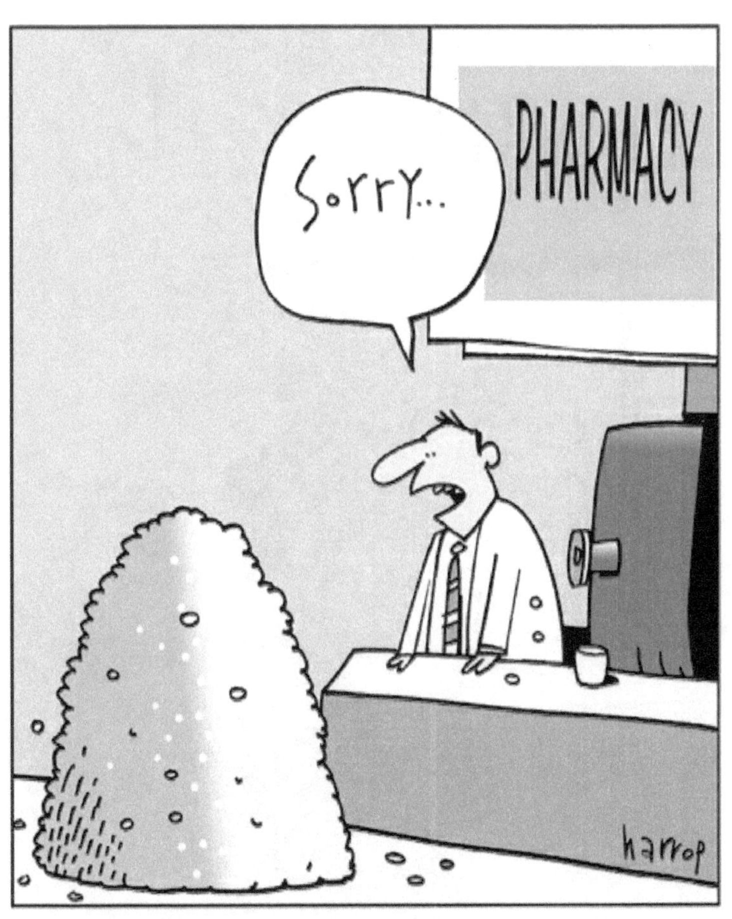

The first robotic pill-dispensing machine still had a few bugs to be worked out.

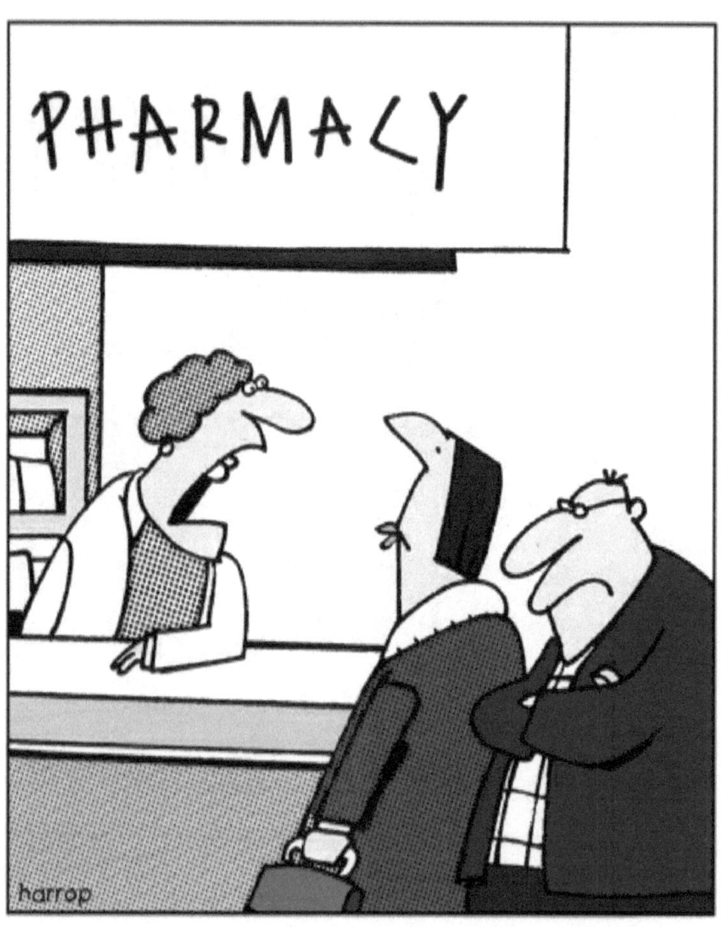

I'm sorry - but to prescribe something for a
'pain in the butt' - it has to be your own!

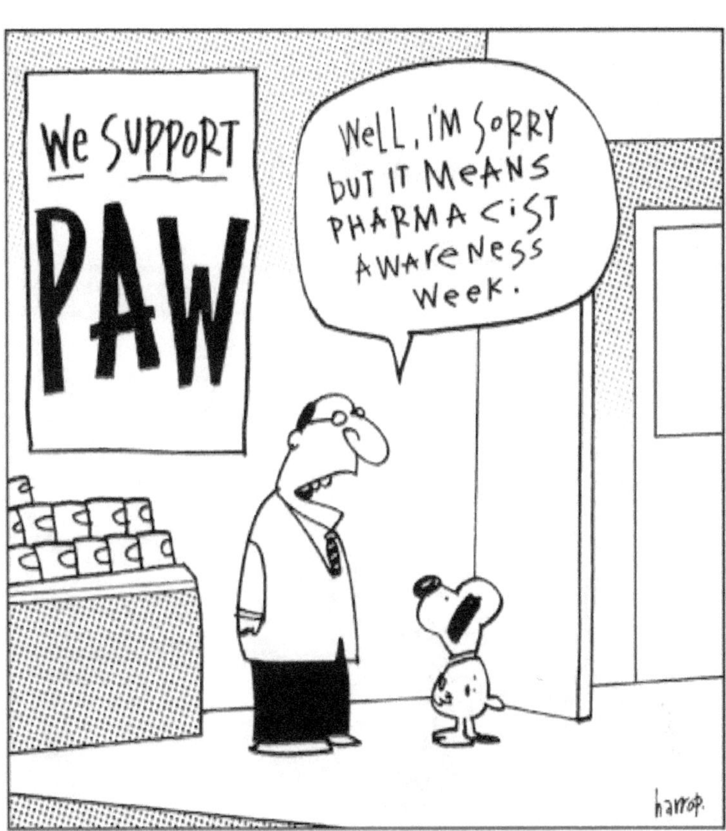

We SUPPORT
PAW
WELL, I'M SORRY
but IT MEANS
PHARMACiST
AWARENESS
WeeK.
harrop.

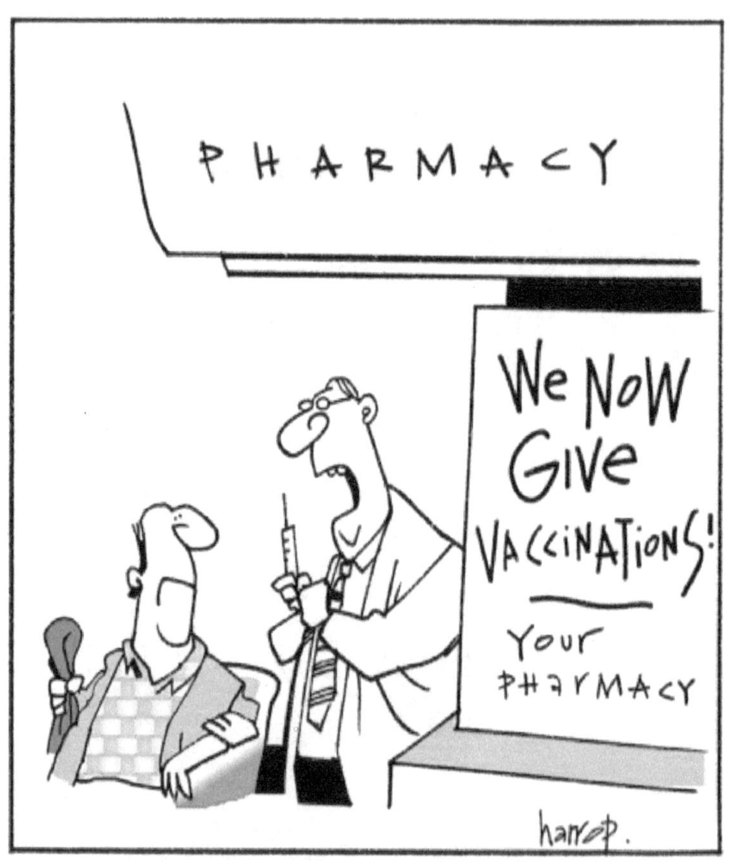

**Before I start ... remember needling ME
about my golf scores?**

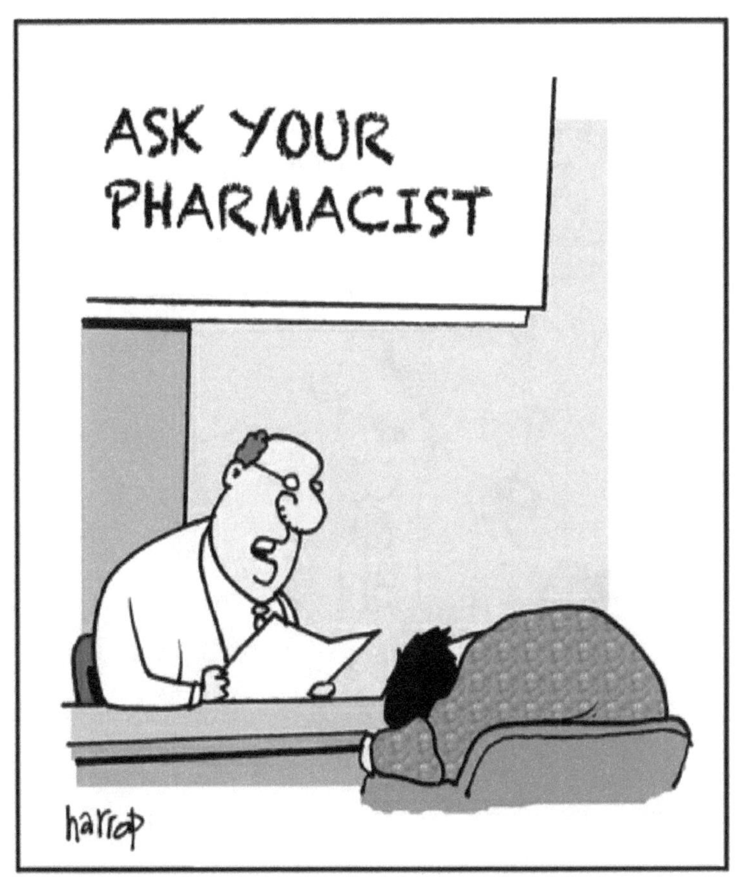

**Frankly, I think you're overdoing it
on the sleep medication .**

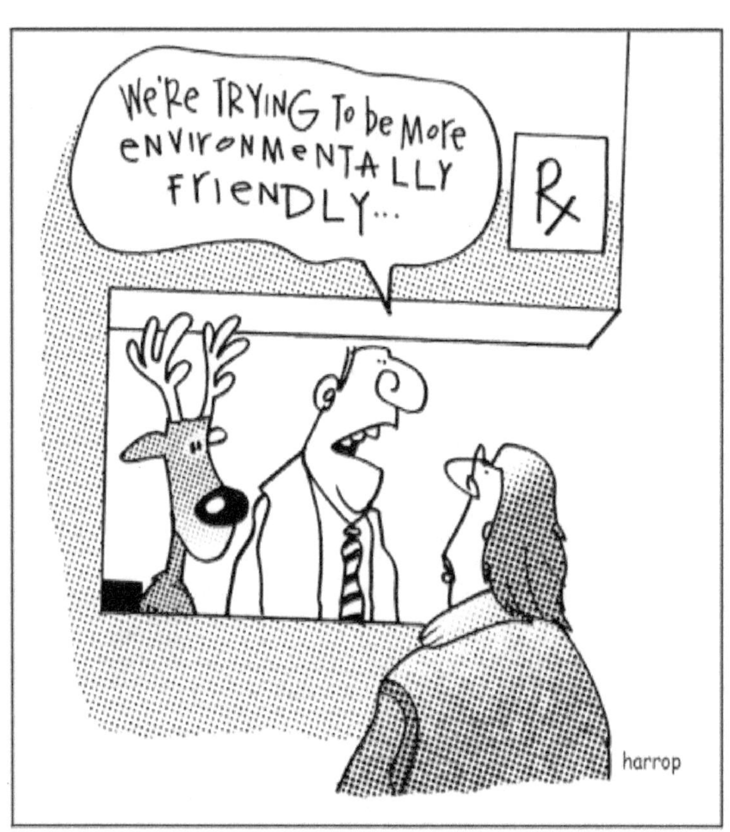

We're TRYING To be More
eNVironMeNTALLY
FrieNDLY...
Rx
harrop

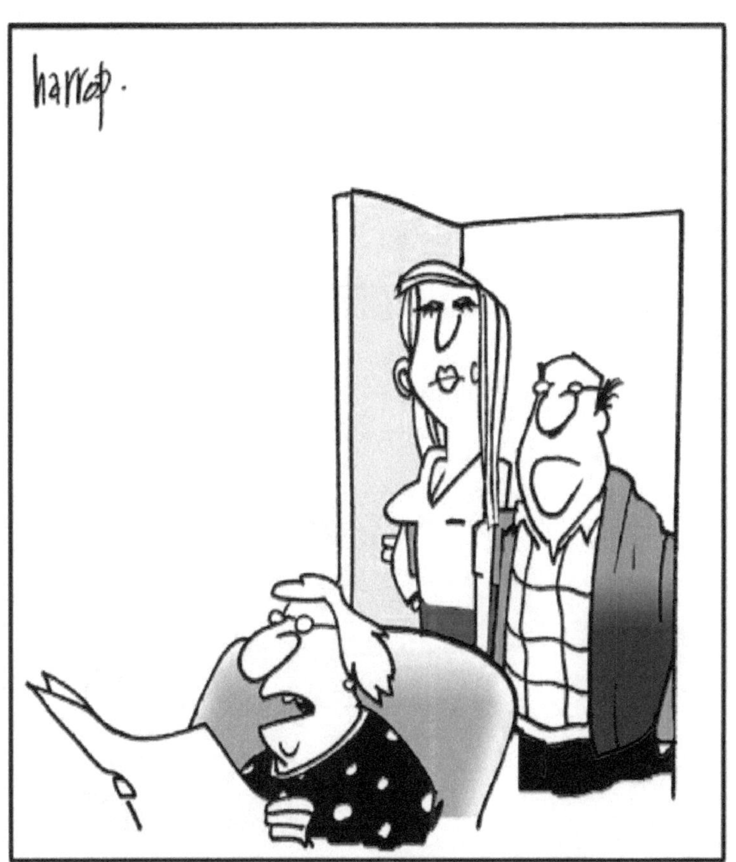

OK - if you're not going for the nicotine replacement therapies, how are you going to take your mind off cigarettes?

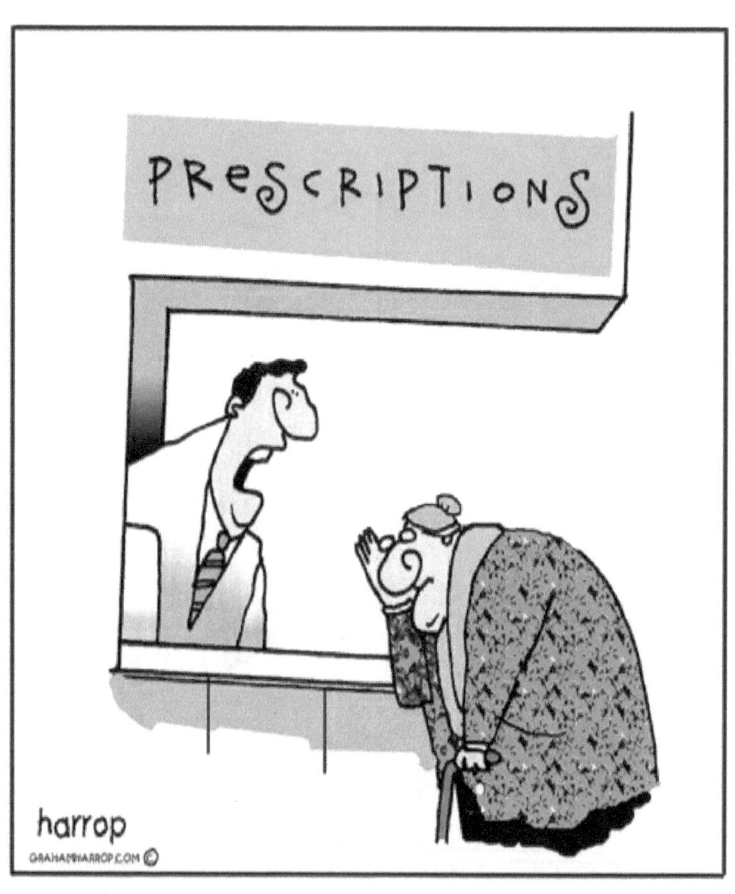

I SAID: 'WILL YOU BE OPERATING
ANY HEAVY MACHINERY?'

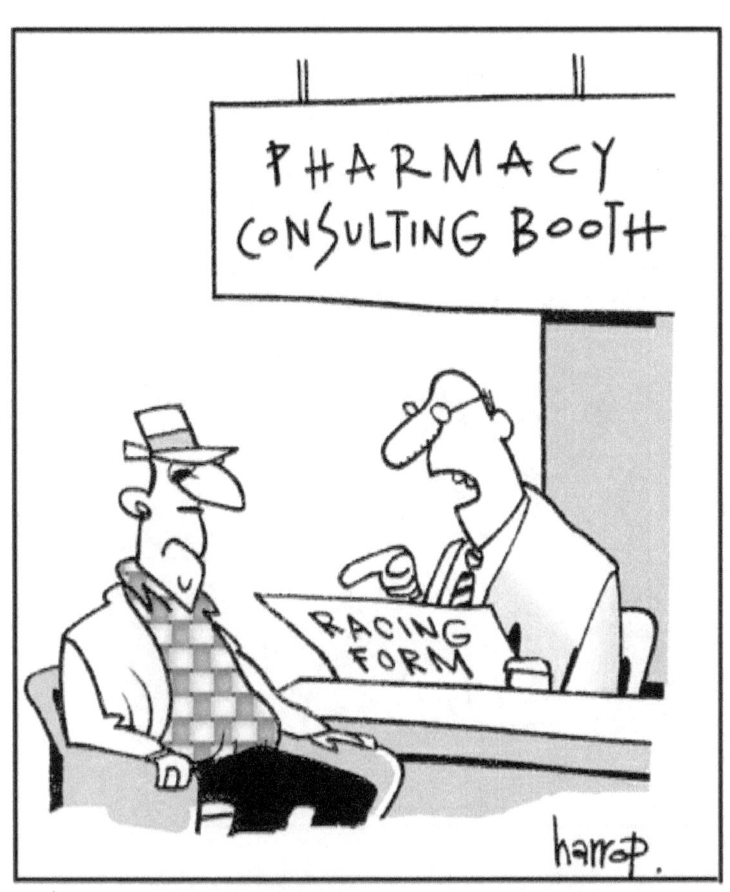

I usually just give advice on prescriptions,
but since you ask, I'm going to say:
'Dancing Boy' in the fourth!

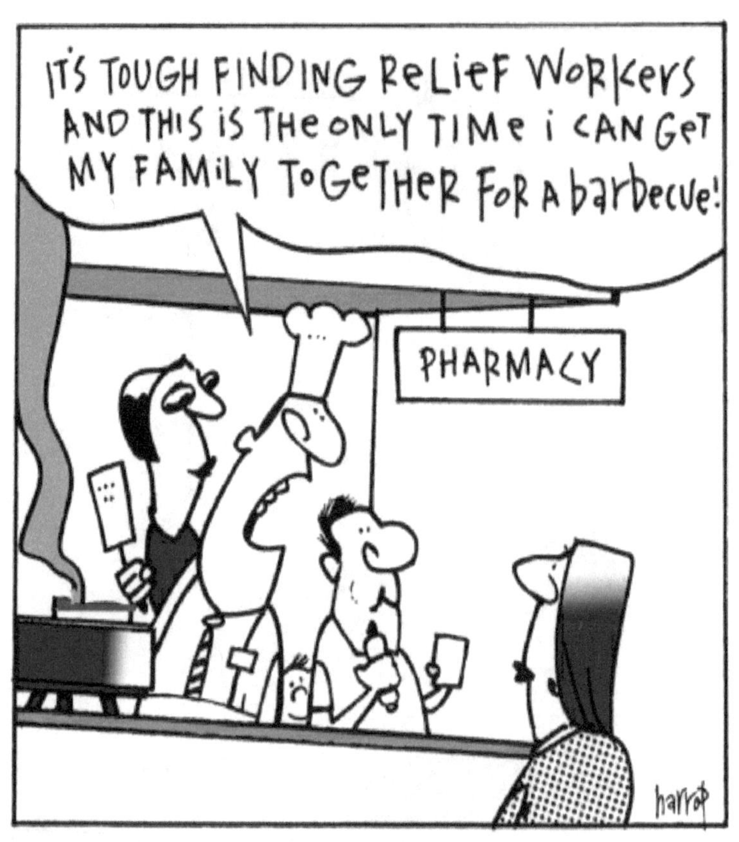

IT'S TOUGH FINDING RELIEF WORKERS AND THIS IS THE ONLY TIME i CAN GET MY FAMILY TOGETHER FOR A barbecue!
PHARMACY
harrop

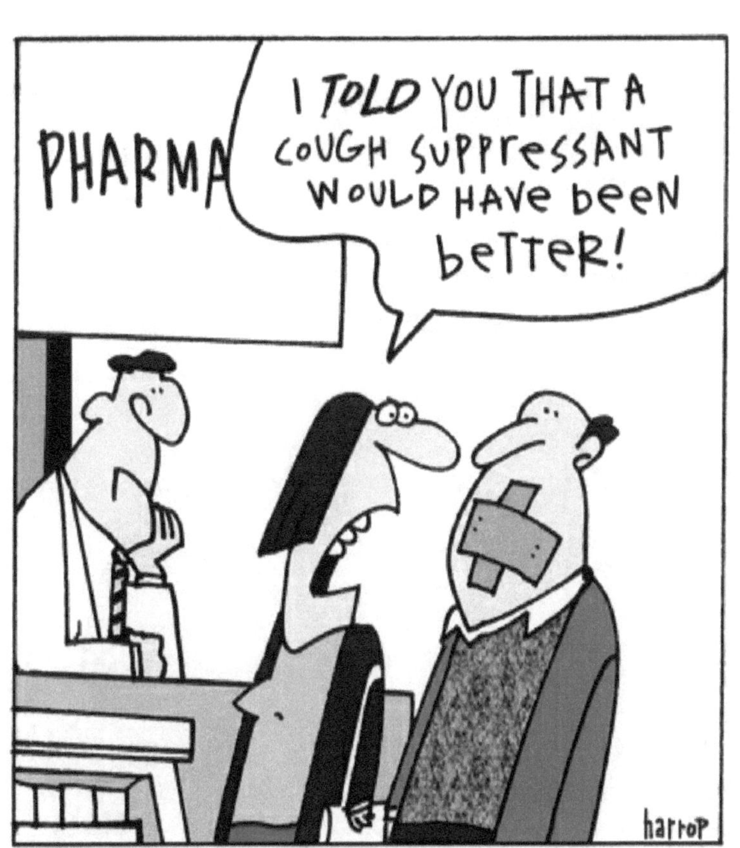

PHARMA
I TOLD YOU THAT A COUGH SUPPRESSANT WOULD HAVE BEEN BETTER!
harrop

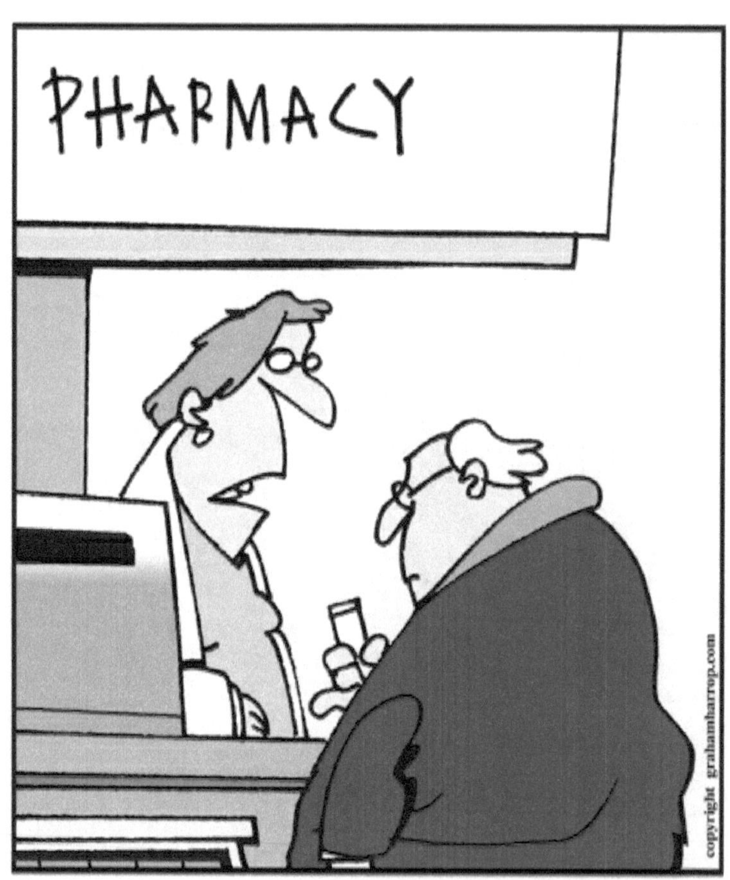

OAD means 'Once a day'
NOT **order a donut!**

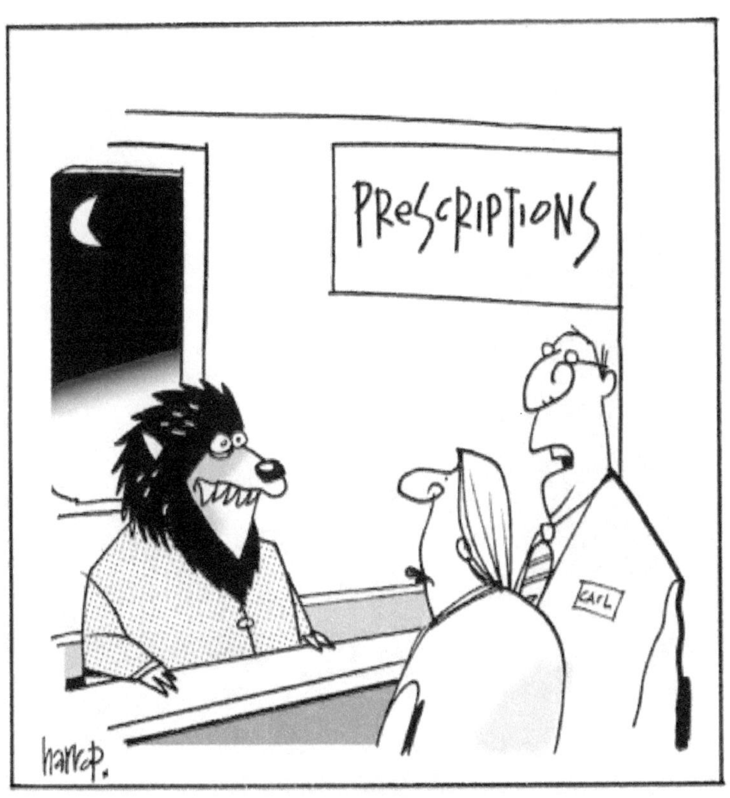

It's all part of being a 24-hour pharmacy...
he wants advice on hair removal.

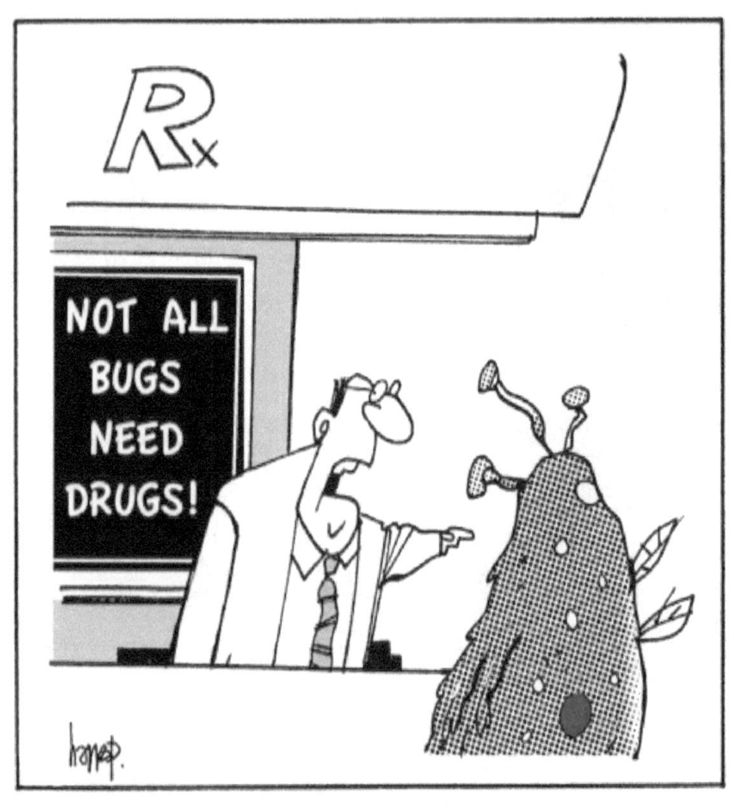

Look - I'm not prepared to debate it...
now *GET OUT!*

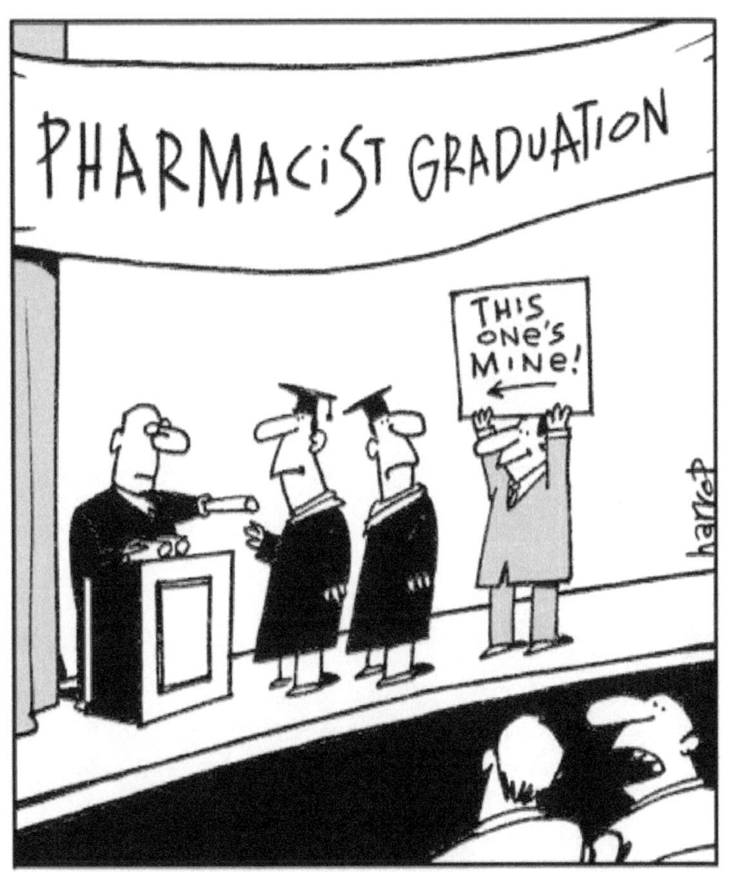

I think it has something to do with the
pharmacist shortage.

9 798732 092929